This book is dedicated
to my friend Rachel
and to all families
whose lives have been
disrupted by cancer.

May your flowers continue to blossom.

Published by: Canyon Beach Visual Communications
2026 Print on Demand Edition, English Version

Authored by Neyal J. Ammary-Risch and Illustrated by Christopher Risch

For more information about the book or to contact the author or illustrator visit:
www.canyonbeach.com/books/inmommysgarden

ISBN: 978-0-9754221-0-6

In Mommy's Garden

A Book to Help Explain Cancer to Young Children

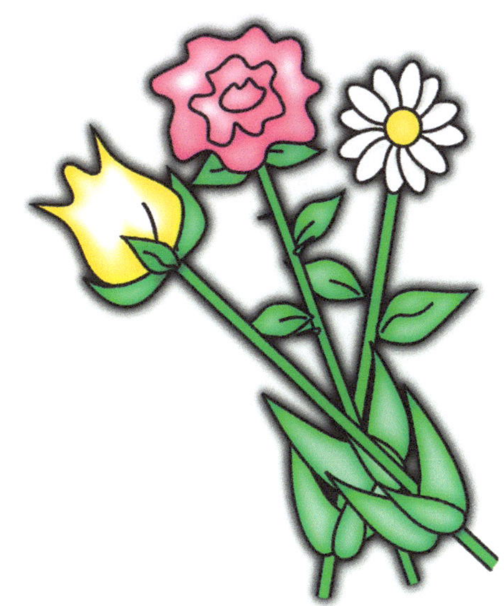

Written By:
Neyal J. Ammary-Risch

Illustrated By:
Christopher Risch

This is my Mommy. She has an illness.
It's called cancer.

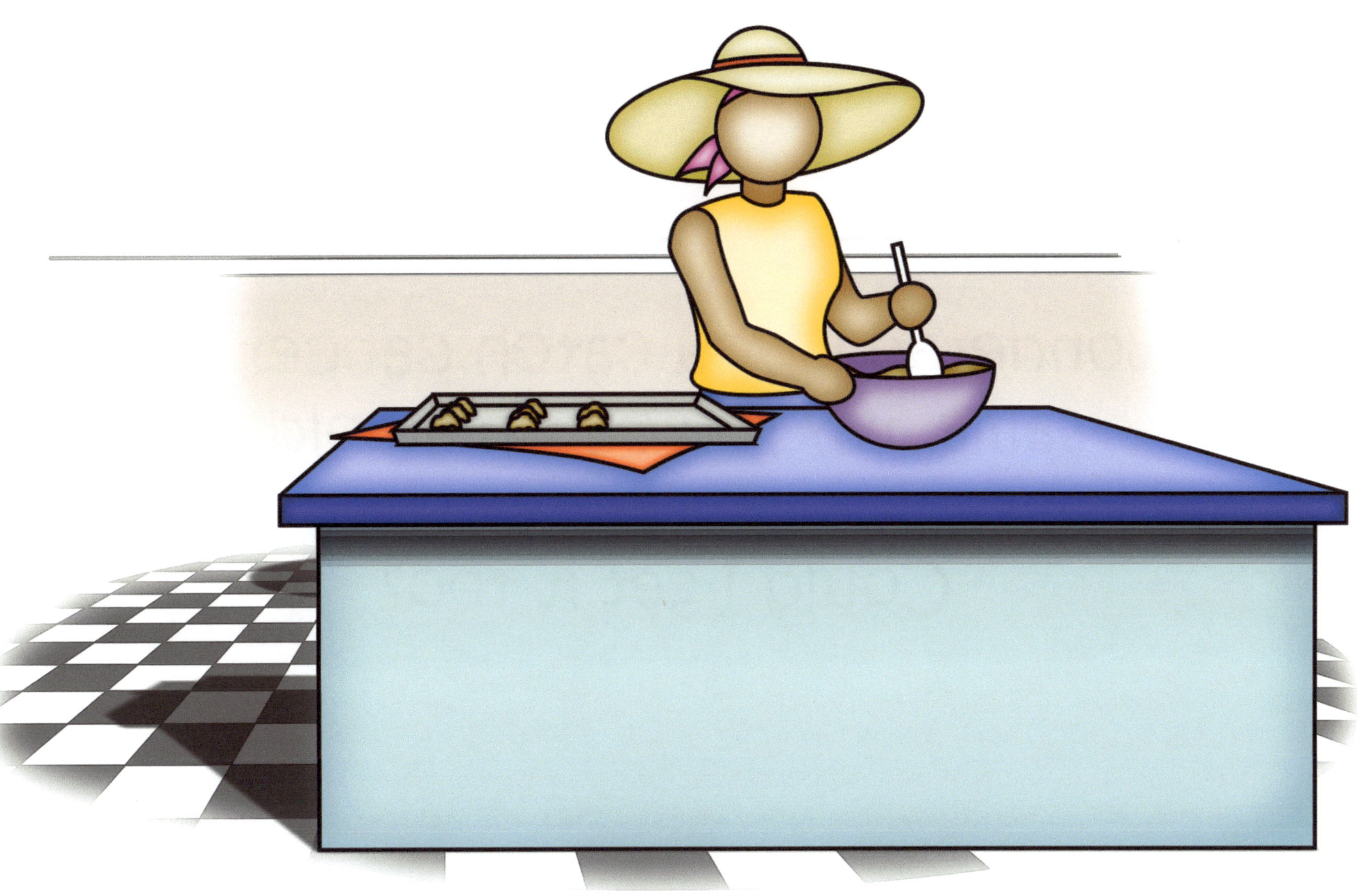

I wondered if you catch cancer the
same way you catch a cold.

Could I get it too?

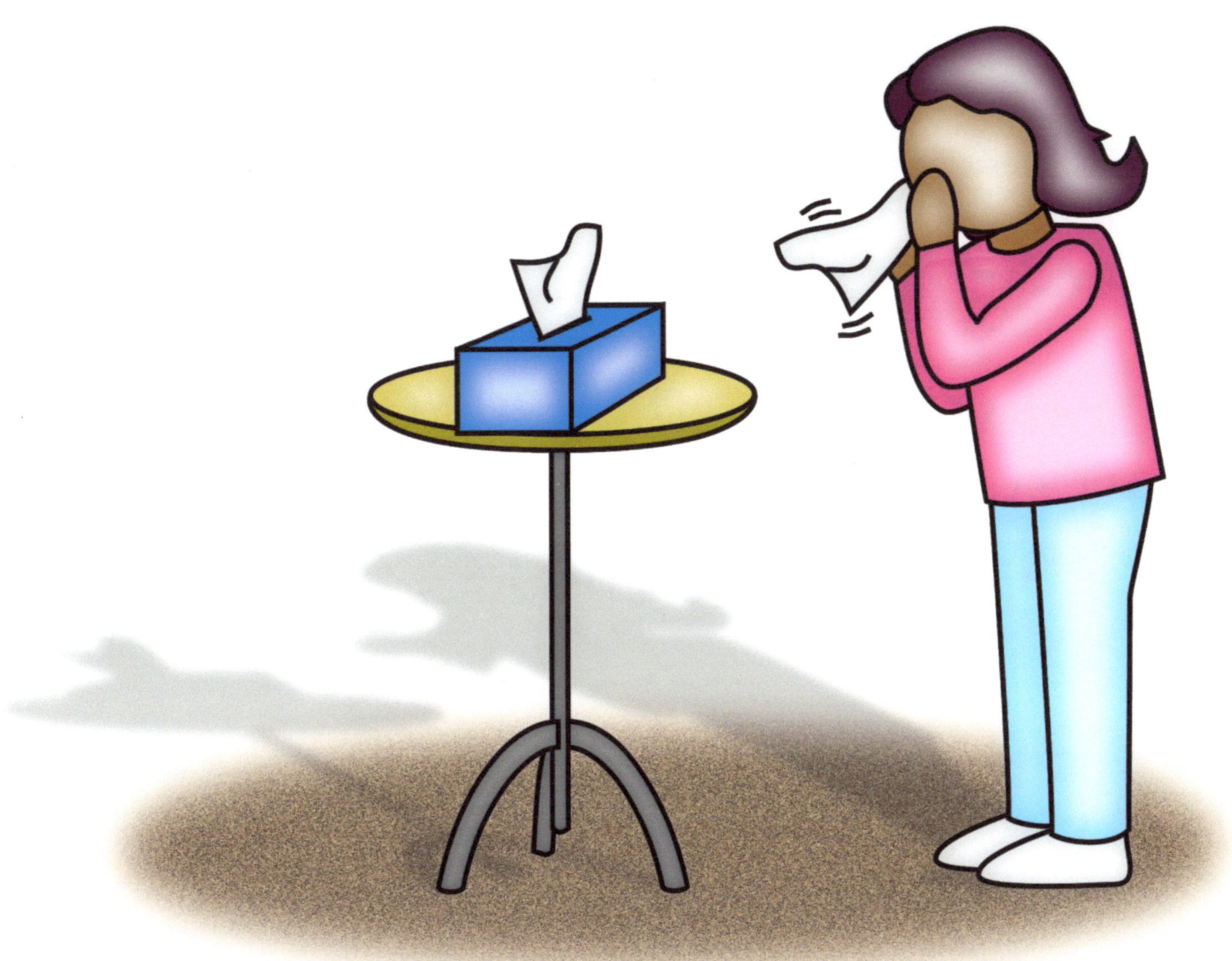

But Mommy told me you can't catch it from anyone else and you can't make anyone get cancer.

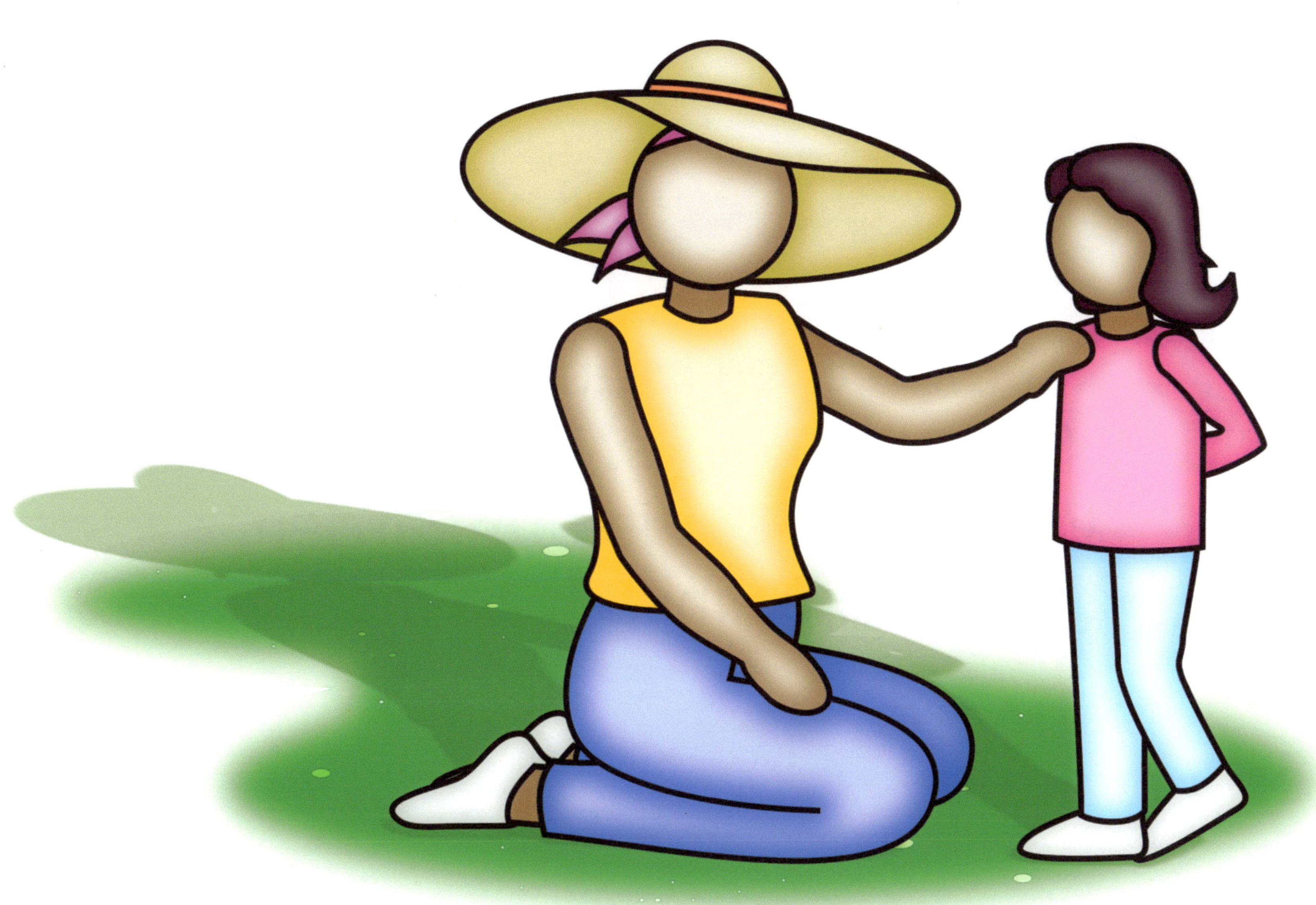

I didn't really understand
what cancer was. But one day,
when we were in our garden,
she explained it to me.

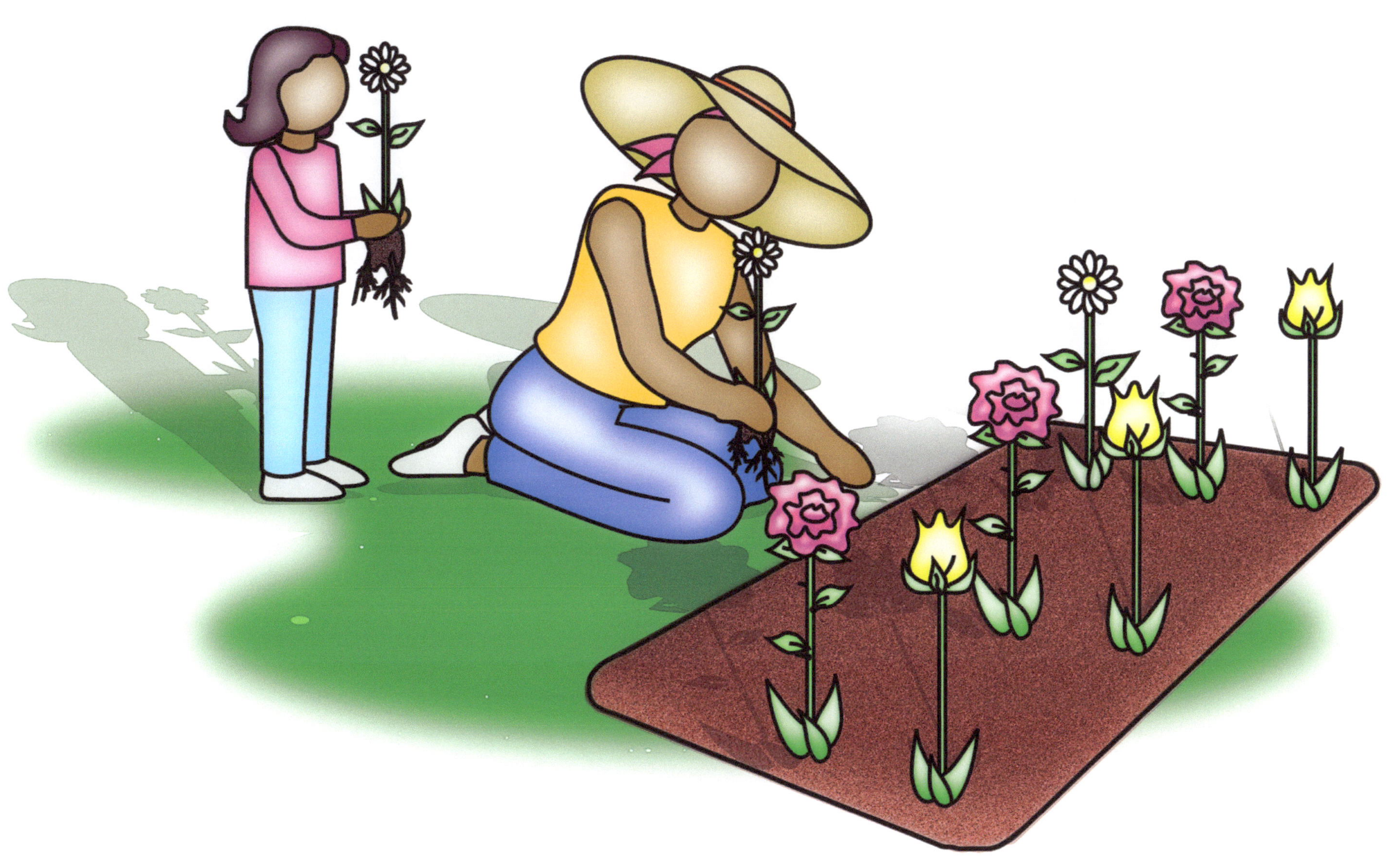

She said that cancer is like the weeds
that grow in our flower garden.

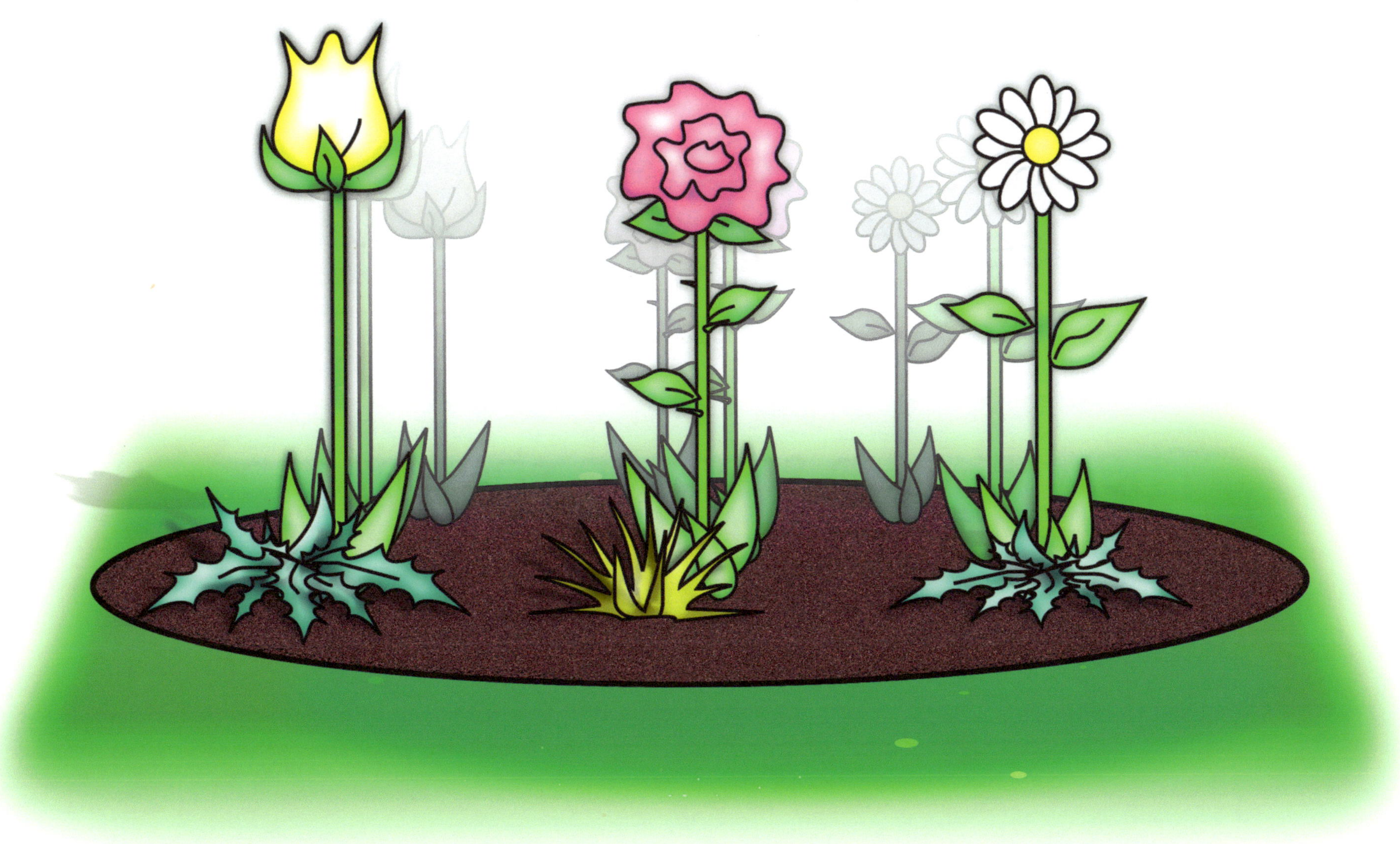

Weeds are bad plants that
hurt the good plants.

They take up space in the garden
and can stop the flowers from
growing tall, colorful, and healthy.

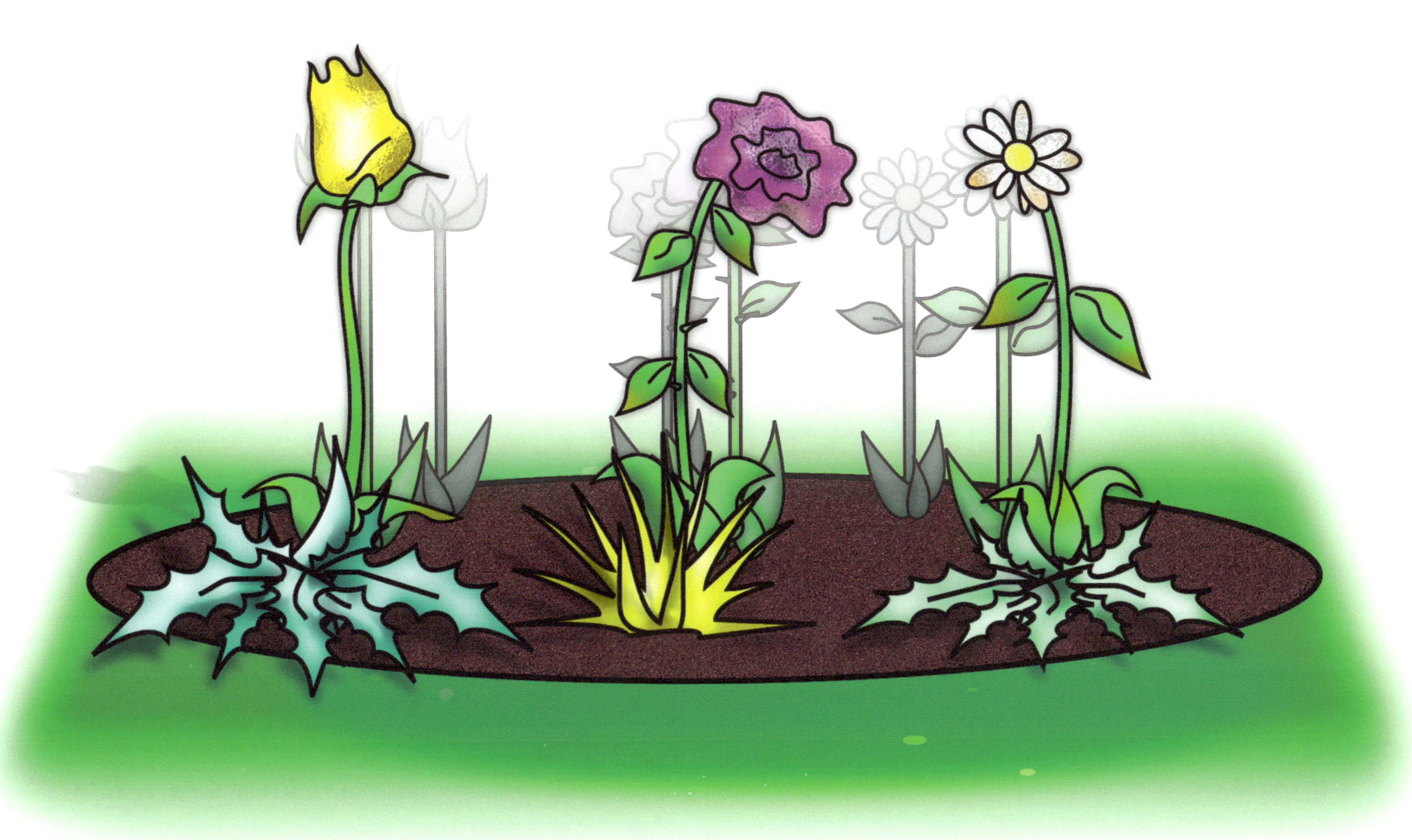

We do things to weeds,
like dig them out or put chemicals
on them so they stop growing.

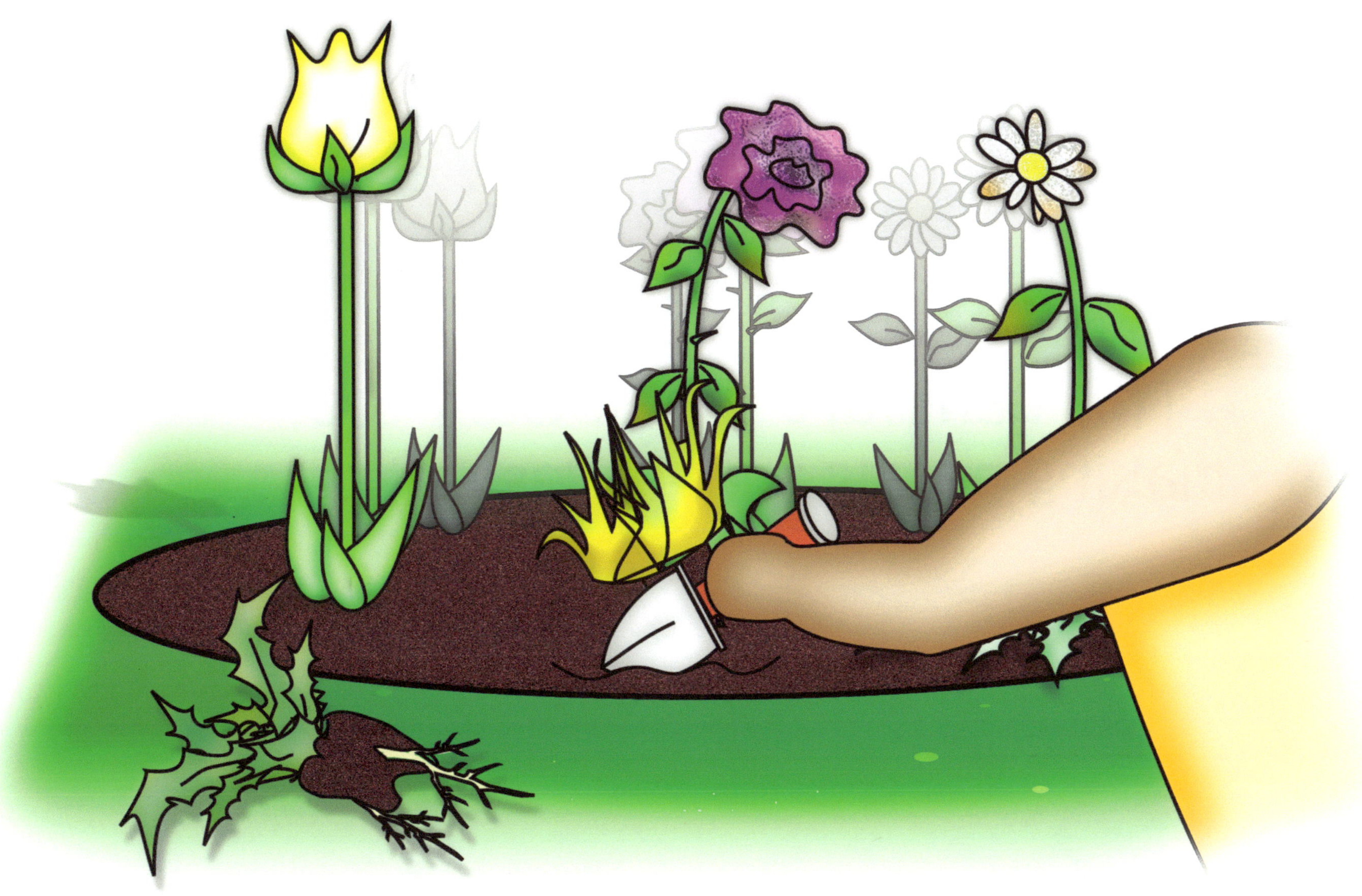

This can hurt the flowers too,
making petals and leaves fall off.

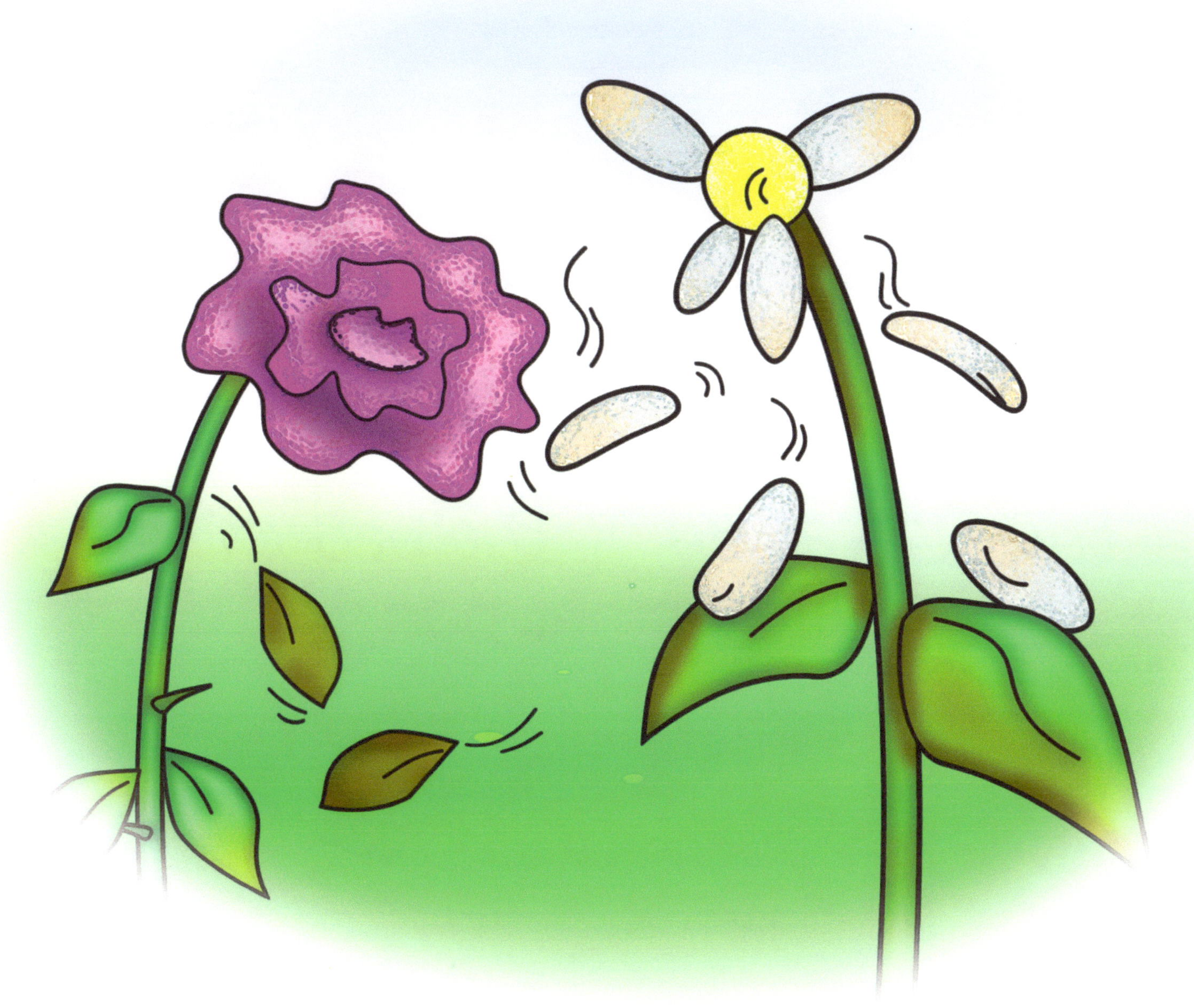

Mommy said the medicine she
takes works the same way.

It tries to get rid of the bad things
growing in her body.

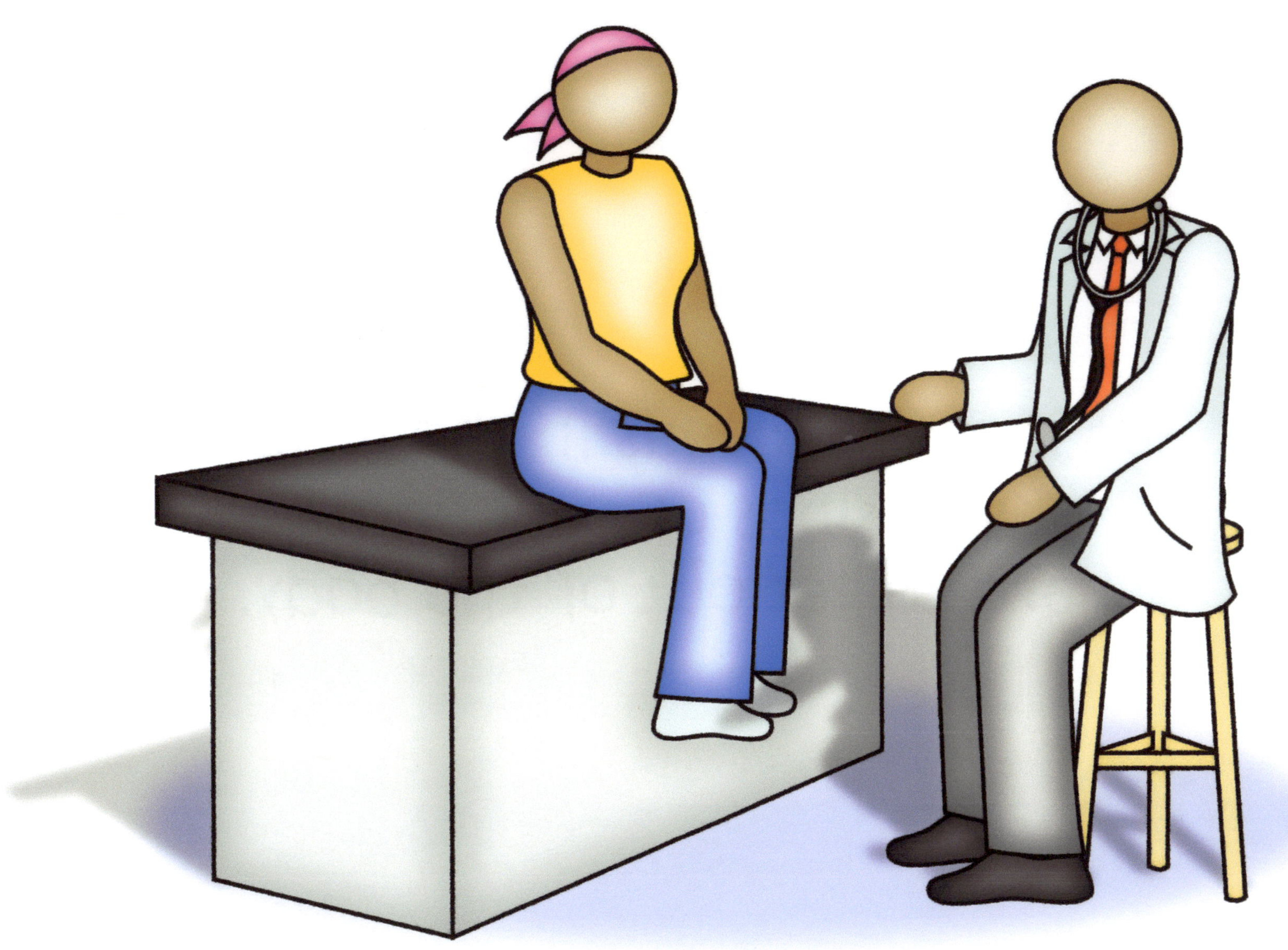

But just like weeds in the ground,
some kinds of cancer are
hard to get out of the body.

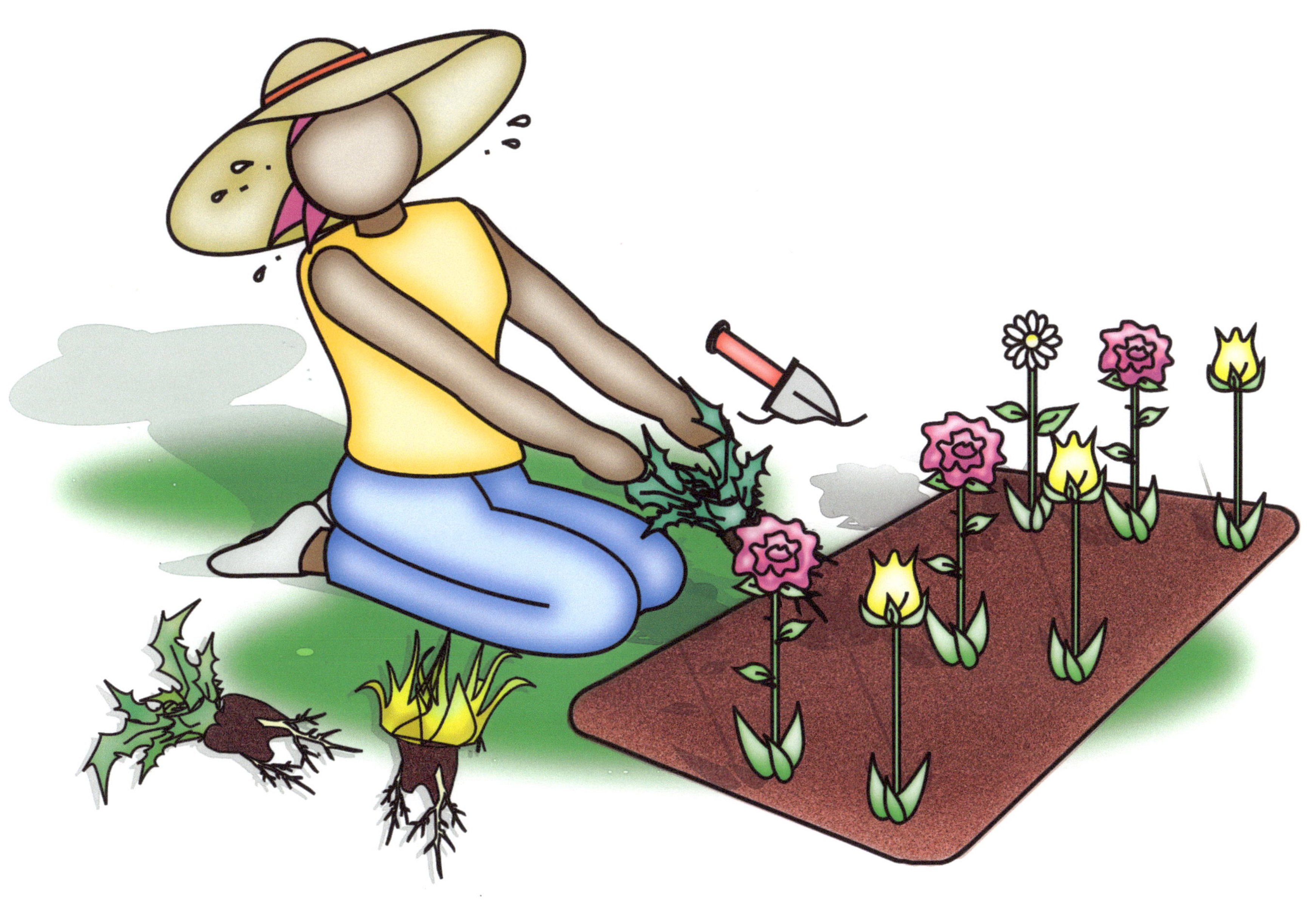

That's why some days Mommy
feels really sick and tired.

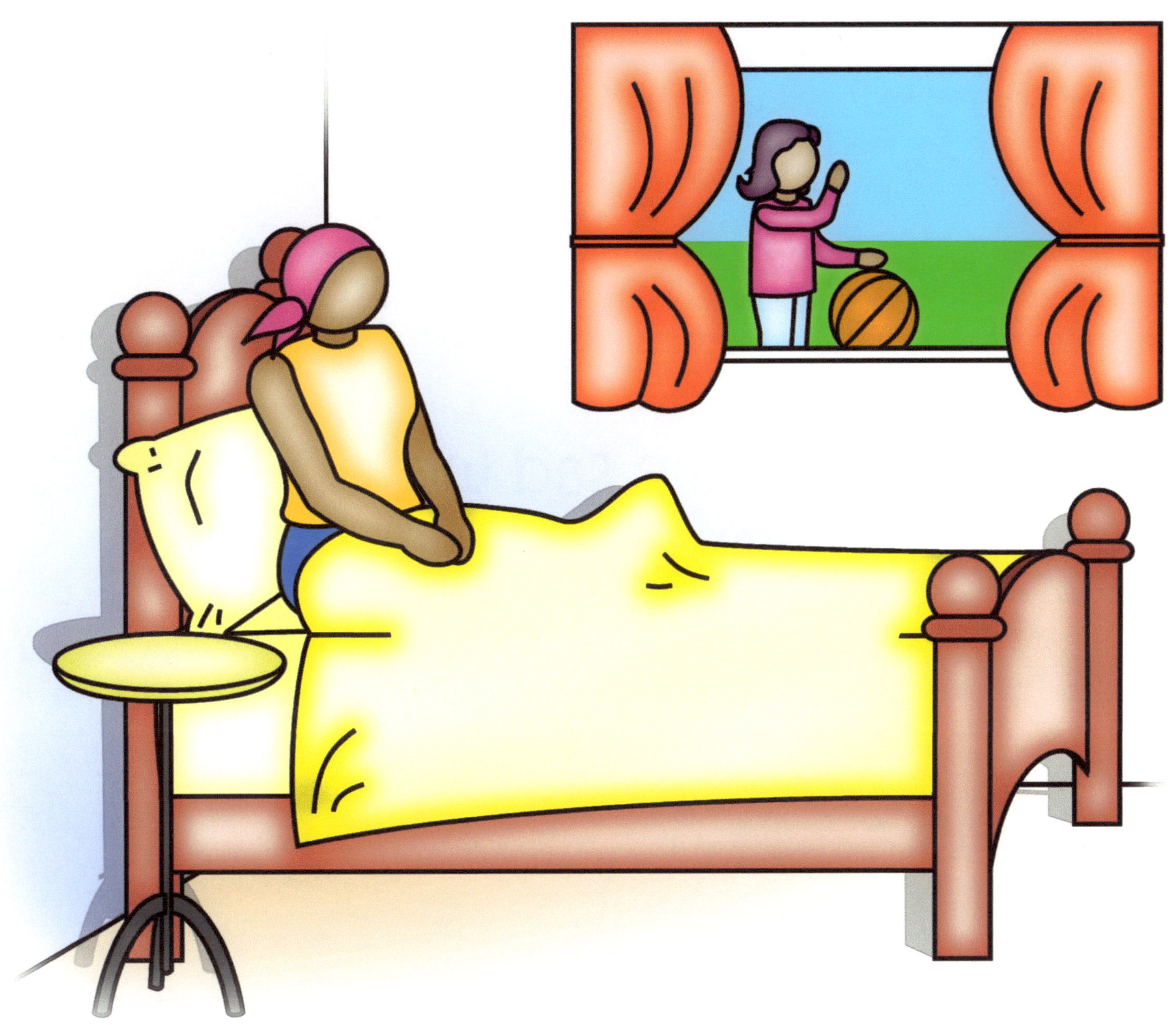

This makes me sad when I want
her to play outside with me.

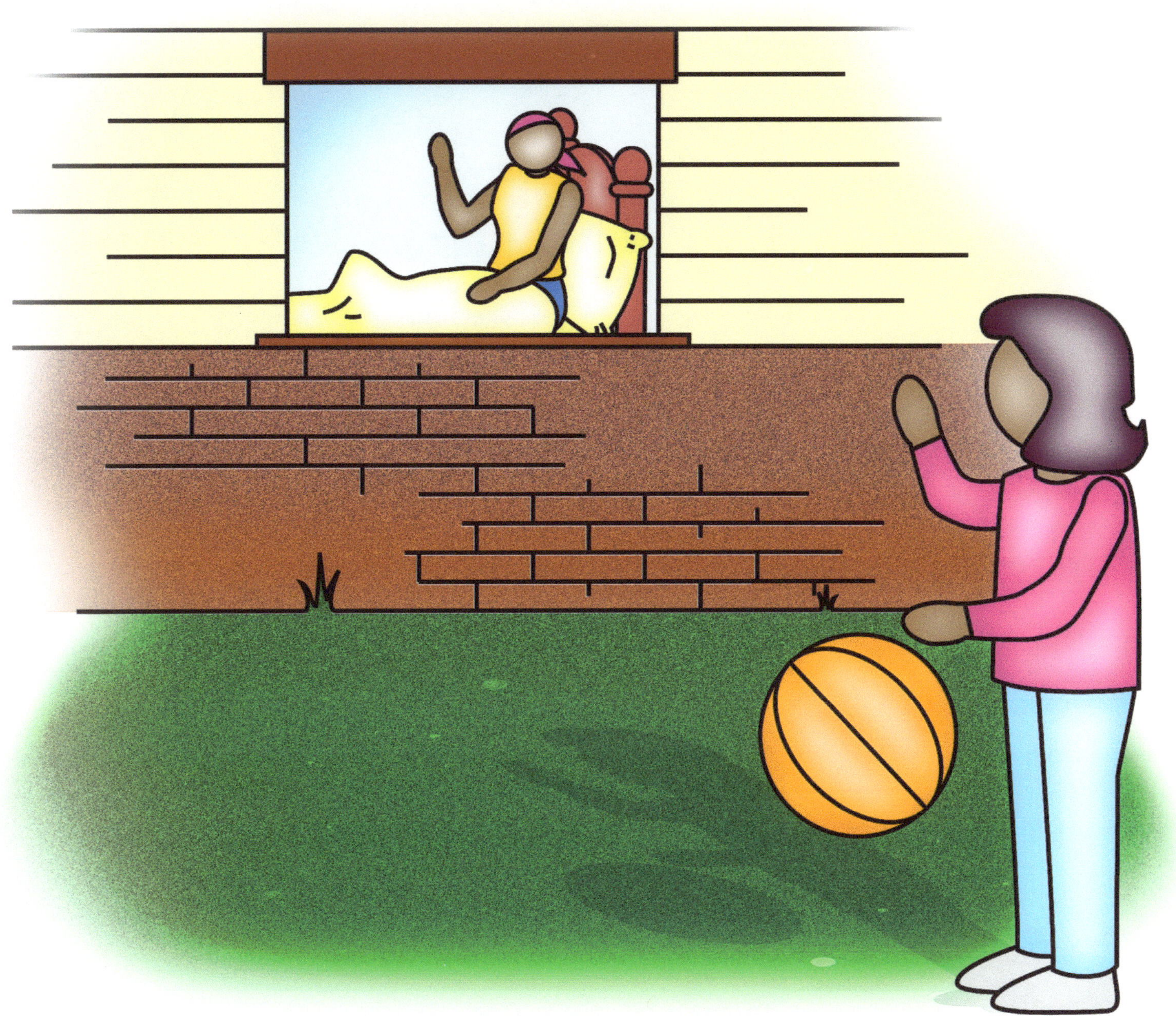

It makes her sad too.

Sometimes she cries. So do I.

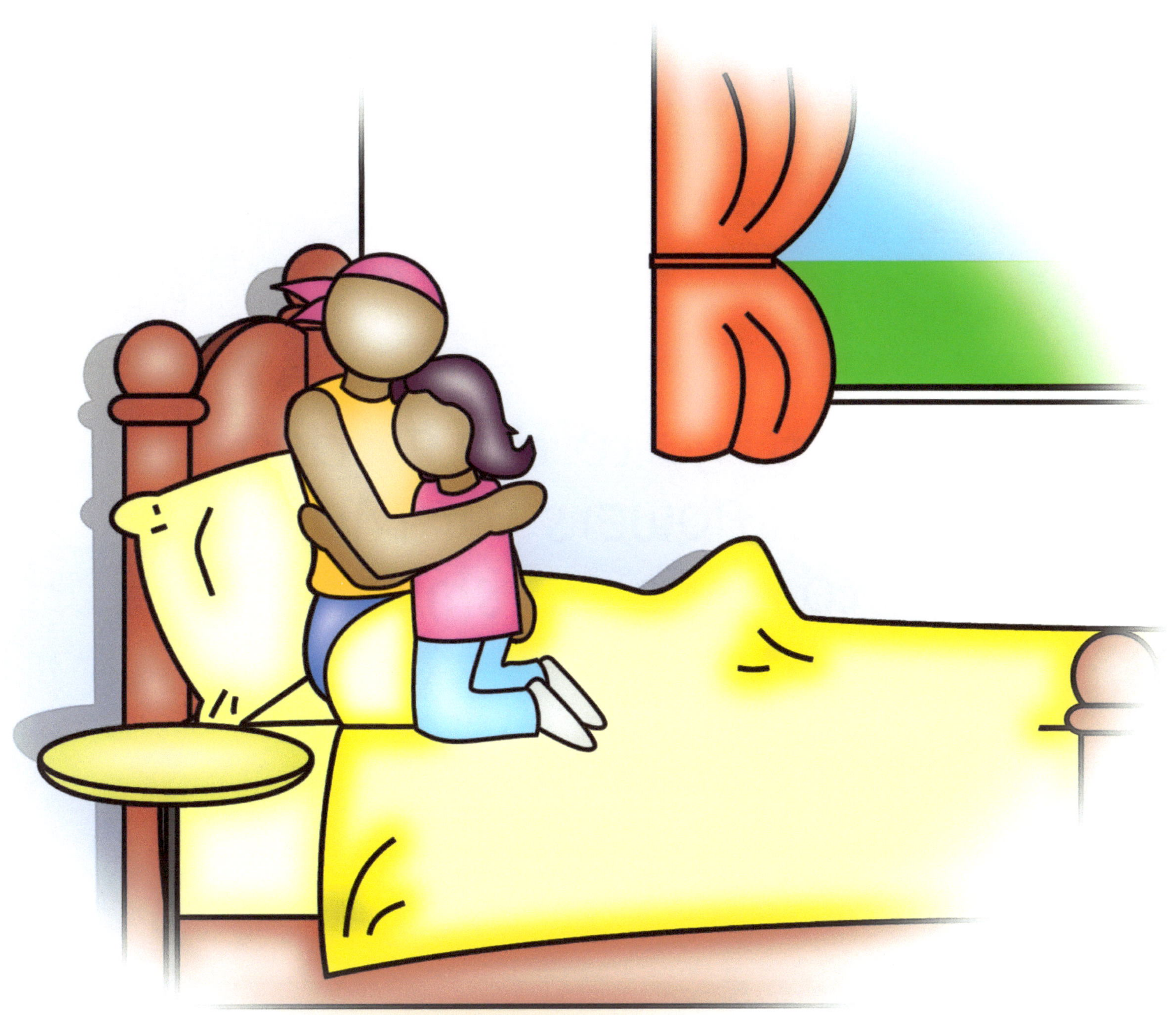

I like to go to the garden
and pick flowers for Mommy
to make her smile.

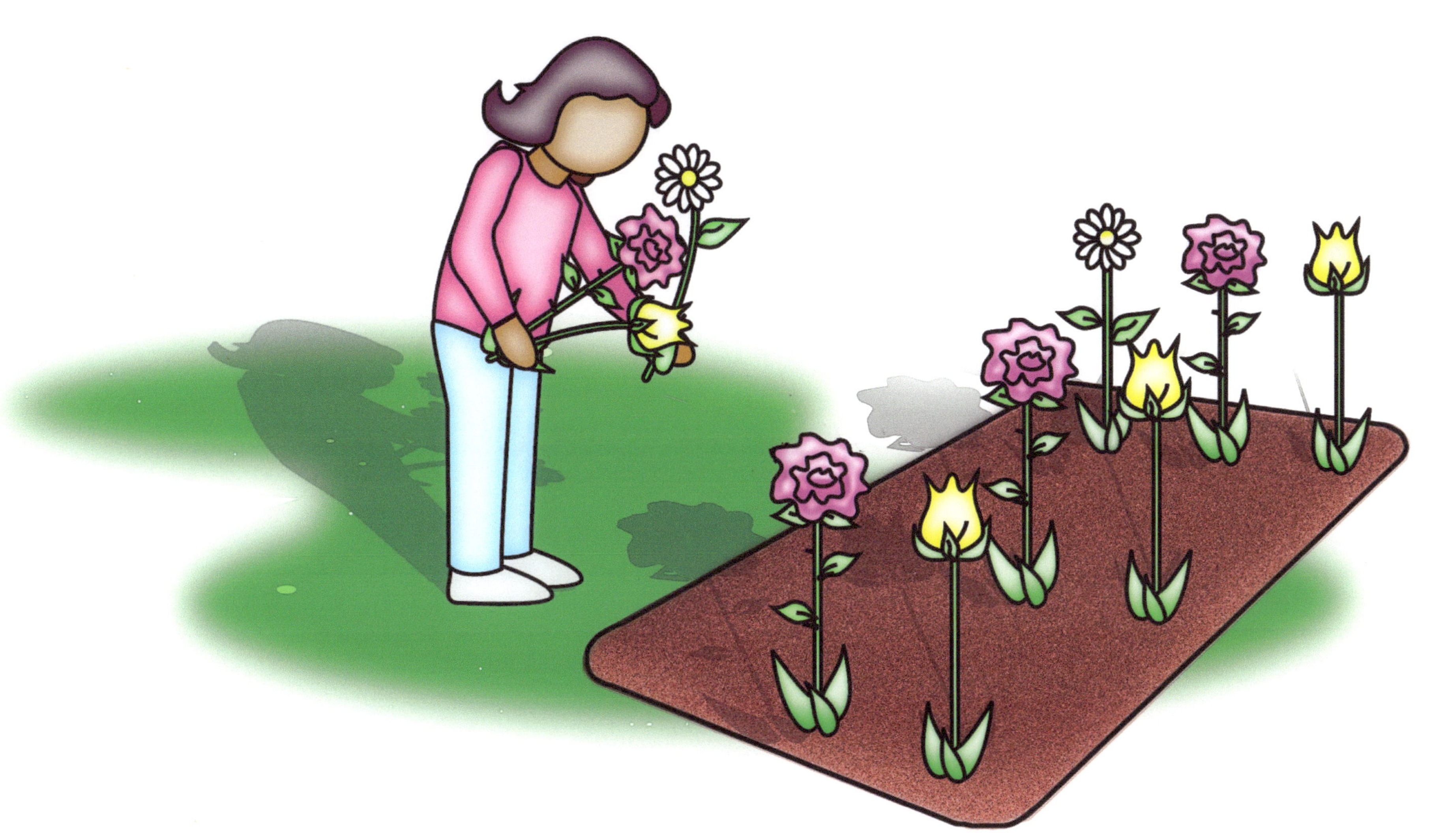

Even with weeds in the garden,
flowers can still be beautiful.

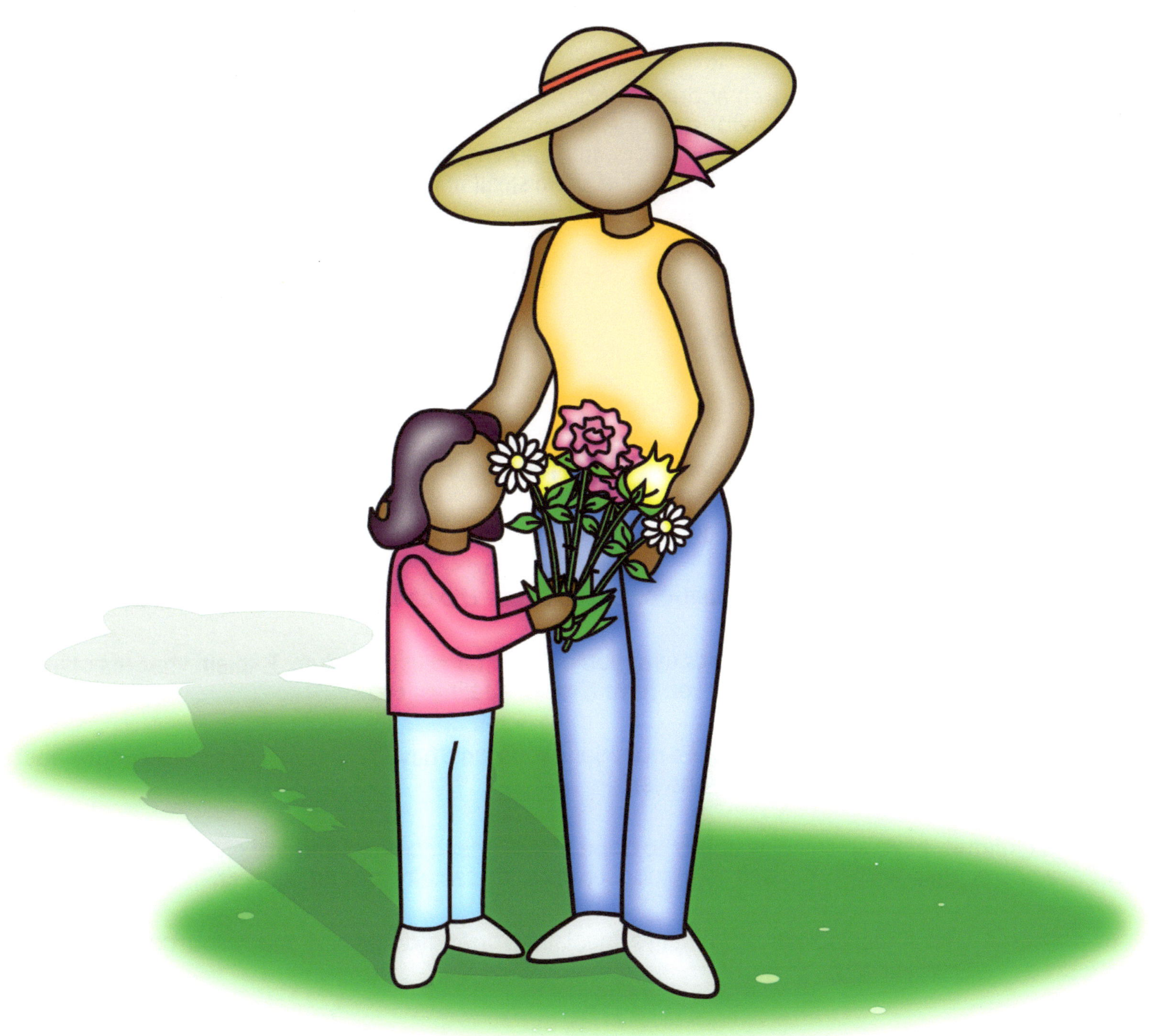

Tips for Talking to Young Children about Cancer

Adults may be reluctant to talk to children about a cancer diagnosis, but being open and honest helps demystify cancer and also helps children feel less anxious. Young children do not need a lot of detailed information. Being truthful about your cancer, its treatment and effects, in a way that is age appropriate, is important for your child's mental well-being. It's best to be honest and give them small amounts of information at a time and in words that are easy for them to understand.

In Mommy's Garden can help you start a conversation with children about cancer. Here are some additional tips:

- Tell them the name of the type of cancer.

- Show them the part of the body where the cancer is.

- Discuss how the cancer will be treated and any side effects, such as hair loss, weight loss, vomiting or fatigue.

- Explain how their lives will be affected and assure them they will still be taken care of.

- Reassure them there's nothing they thought or did to cause the cancer and that they cannot catch it.

- Encourage children to share their feelings with you or another trusted adult. Explain that it's okay to have a wide range of feelings. Let them know you have a lot of feelings, too.

- Don't be afraid to answer "I don't know" to questions you don't have an answer to or aren't sure how to answer. Tell them you'll try to find an answer.

- Be honest. Children have an amazing ability to cope if they feel included and are given support; even sad truths are better than anxiety caused by misconceptions, uncertainties and secrets.

Talk to your doctor, nurse, social worker or child life specialist for additional tips and resources to help your family cope with a cancer diagnosis.

All gardens are beautiful. Draw and color your own garden.

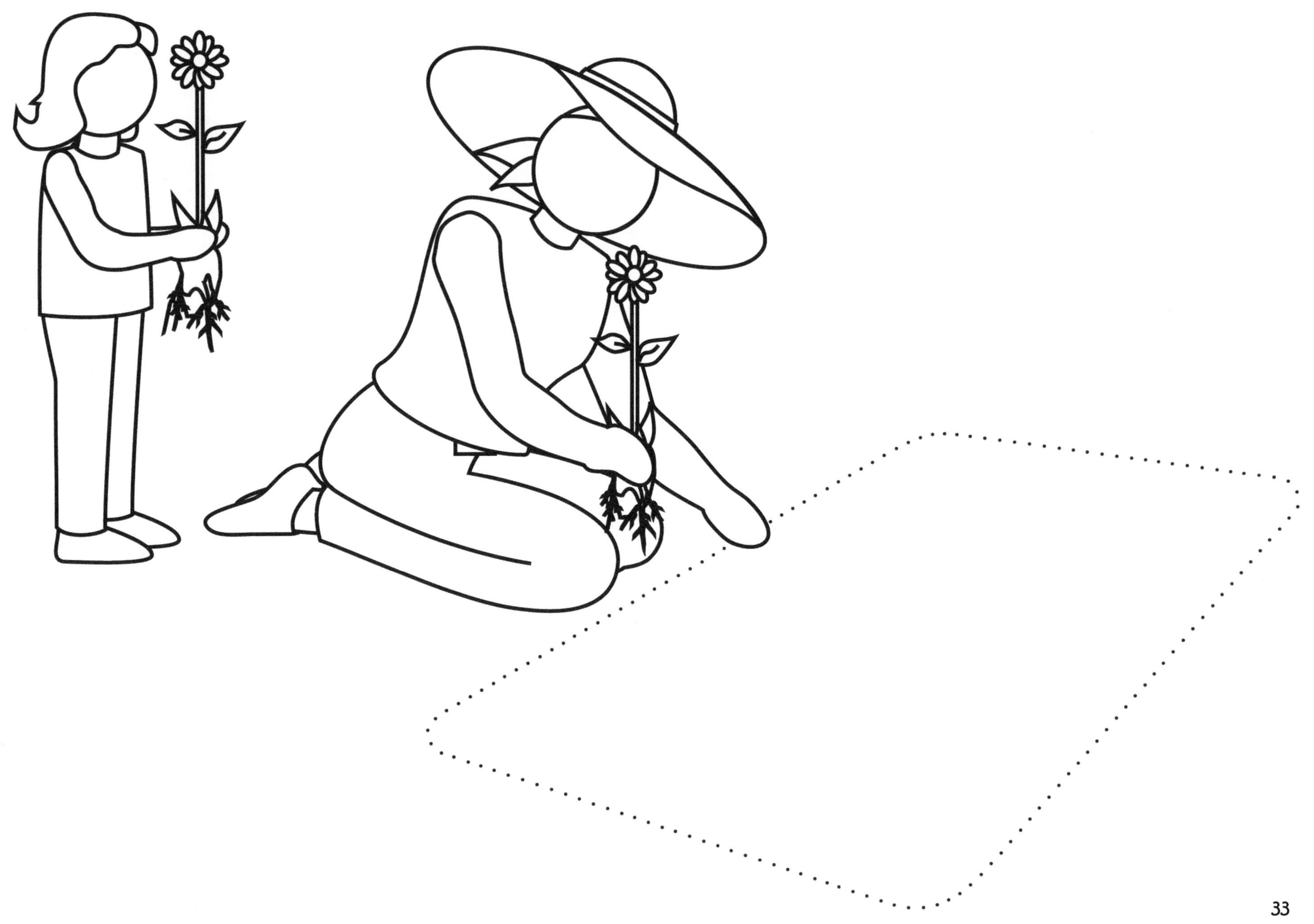

Draw a picture to make your loved one with cancer smile.